Creative
Walking
for Physical Fitness

5

Creative Walking for Physical Fitness

HARRY J. JOHNSON, M. D., *with RALPH BASS*

Photographs by Elizabeth Wilcox

GROSSET & DUNLAP
A NATIONAL GENERAL COMPANY
Publishers • New York

In recent years the walker in the city and in the country as well has encountered a previously non-existent hazard: pollution. In the cities the very air he breathes is frequently semi-poisonous, while the streams of the countryside flow with disgusting sludge. Thus, all too often the joy of walking is replaced by dismay and even fear. Belatedly, our national leaders as well as our average citizens have awakened to the menace of a contaminated land. It will take every ounce of their determination to halt the spreading horror.

It is because we appreciate the enormous nature of their task that we dedicate this book to the men and women who are fighting to keep America clean. Unless this fight is won, our costly efforts to help peoples in other parts of the globe will be a tragic irony.

DR. HARRY J. JOHNSON

Contents

Introduction

Over a long medical career I have had ample opportunity to observe that most people like to follow the course of least resistance. At the Life Extension Institute we have grown used to seeing people whose health problems have arisen largely out of their own inertia. Physical laziness gives rise to mental laziness, and the day soon comes when they begin to wonder why life seems so unsatisfactory.

These people are only half alive—if that. Unfortunately, we doctors often have to settle for *keeping* them half alive. And sometimes even this presents a problem. One recent study of 110,000 adults revealed that men classified as "least active" physically are four times more likely to die of a heart attack than the "moderately active." And they are twice as prone to a first heart attack.

When we consider that there are about half a million deaths from coronary heart disease in this country every year—four out of five of them among men—we begin to visualize the dimensions of the problem.

Although this and similar findings have been given wide publicity, the man who says he never stands when he can sit and never sits when he can lie down is usually only half joking. That is why

9

so many theoretically useful exercise devices and machines—and they grow in number and ingenuity every month—usually end up rusting away in sheds and closets. Pick up one of the "for sale or exchange" publications that circulate in the suburbs and you will get an inkling of just how many people decide that the equipment is not working out. Or, perhaps more accurately, that *they* are not working out.

This all-too-human trait of taking it easy is not confined to the use of machines. Many men and women join "Y"s and other gymnasiums and health clubs for swimming, calisthenics, and so on. They sincerely mean to go at least once a week, and yet one day it dawns on them that their most recent use of the undeniably excellent facilities dates back several months. At this point they usually shrug their shoulders and forget the whole thing.

The number of joggers is dwindling for much the same reason: the routine of changing into suitable clothes and taking to the road at appropriate hours—usually before or after work and on weekends—disenchants many who start with great enthusiasm.

People who are "hooked" on games like tennis usually manage to play regularly. Yet tennis and other vigorous sports sometimes involve a little danger particularly, to the previously sedentary individual.

There is no lack of "health books," but this one is written with a special purpose. That purpose is to convey my deep conviction that there is one exercise—plain, old-fashioned walking—that is completely beneficial and convenient, and at the same time risk-free. I have seen such spectacular results from it that I do not hesitate to "go overboard" as a zealot or missionary or whatever other label may be affixed.

And because I believe that walking is *essential* to the health I will go so far as to urge all of you to *Walk For Your Life*.

Harry J. Johnson, M.D.

Introduction

The real beginning of my association with Dr. Harry Johnson and this book involves quite a few people. Some were relatives, some friends, some comparative strangers. Yet they had one thing in common—their eyes seemed to dwell for longer and longer periods on my midsection. After a while, I got the idea. There was more and more midsection to look at.

The sad fact was that I had gone from a vigorous youth to a somewhat less so early manhood to a listless and—to put it bluntly —fat middle age. And the strange thing about it was that I hadn't really noticed. True, I wheezed a little when I climbed stairs, and the one time I got into a pick-up basketball game I lasted just ten seconds before I felt the cold hand of death beckoning in my direction.

As a writer on medical subjects I had read most of the books on physical fitness. But I still drove the five blocks to pick up the newspaper and rolls every morning. It was not until I met Dr. Johnson who is a very persuasive man that I began to see the light and use my feet. After a year of walking—with only occasional backsliding—I feel a decade younger and find people looking at my face instead of at my abdomen.

In any event, I am proud to be associated with Dr. Johnson in the making of this book. I hope *Creative Walking* will remind people that walking is fun and it works wonders for your physical and mental health.

Ralph Bass

11

Creative
Walking
for Physical Fitness

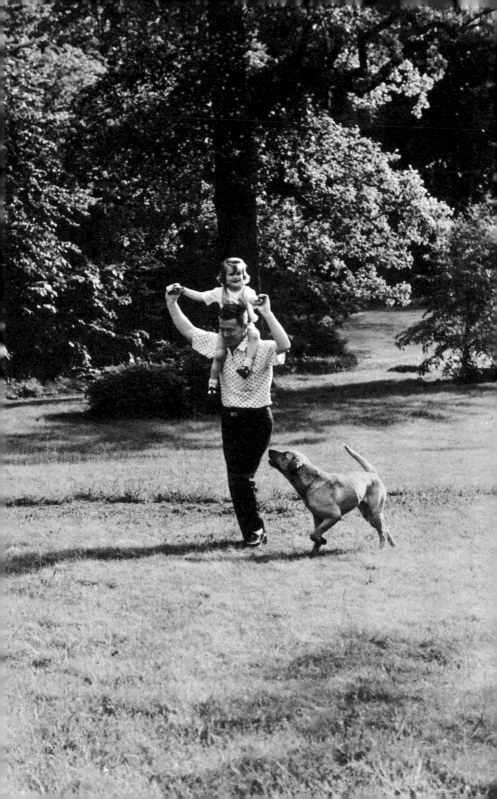

1/Why Walk?

There are many good reasons for walking, some of them more attractive to one type of person than to another. Some find spiritual or esthetic rewards—and these cannot be discounted—but our major emphasis here is on the direct benefit to health as a result of what we may call "creative walking."

Doctors are keenly aware of the flesh and blood reality behind the heart attack statistics. They know that as we grow older the arteries of the heart may narrow—frequently as a result of fatty desposits. These deposits may be due to sluggish circulation, just as silt accumulates in a lazy stream. If we keep our circulation active through the right kind of exercise, we may delay or even prevent this accumulation of debris along the arterial canals.

If the artery *does* narrow and blood has difficulty flowing through the heart, a blood clot or blockage can occur. This is the cause of attack.

When the blockage deprives a section of the heart of the blood it needs, there is still hope. *That hope lies in the body's ability to supply blood to the heart through a collateral blood supply system. And the way to establish this collateral blood supply before a heart attack occurs is through exercise.*

15

THE WAY IT WORKS

How does exercise do this? Somewhat paradoxically, by throwing a burden on the heart over and above its resting capacity. By making the heart work harder, exercise builds up the heart muscle, just as work strengthens any other muscle of the body. At the same time, it helps lay down a "fail-safe" collateral circulation system that can bring blood to the heart during a crisis.

And this is where walking comes in. From long experience we have come to know that it is *mild stress over a long period of time* that can best develop this collateral circulation through the gradual expansion of other branches of arteries in the heart. *Walking supplies exactly the kind of stress that is needed.*

There is still another way in which walking helps our circulation. It builds up the leg muscles that, with their vigorous flexing, press against the veins in the lower part of the body, prodding them into performing their vital function of pumping blood back to the heart. Since this pumping must be done against the force of gravity, the veins need the forceful help that weak leg muscles cannot possibly supply.

BET YOUR LIFE?

It is true, of course, that you may get along, if you are lucky, with coronary circulation that is not up to par. Yet the sword of Damocles is always poised over your head. That is not a situation that makes for carefree living. It will certainly contribute to your peace of mind to know that the "spare" circulation you develop by judicious exercise can provide the armor you need.

The key word is "judicious." You must not be an eager beaver as you develop this collateral circulation. Your exertions may bring about the very thing you are trying to avoid—over-taxing your heart before the collateral circulation is fit to assume part of the load.

That is why walking is the perfect exercise. Involving all parts of the body in its gentle rhythm, it gradually imposes the necessary

16

mild, extra stress on the heart. When the demand is not unreasonable—as in over-vigorous exercise—the heart will respond by developing new life-saving circulation.

That, in a nutshell, is the case for walking. It provides the stress needed to bring about new circulation without ever becoming strenuous enough to cause damage, and it creates strength where strength is needed.

DON'T COMPETE

It is this reasonableness, or moderation, that puts walking in a class by itself as far as exercise is concerned. There is no competitive challenge to lure you into unwise over-exertion. The exercise your walk provides can be mild or vigorous as you choose, based on *your own* recognition of how you feel. After all, you are the best judge. You may take a short walk or a long one, adjusting your pace as you feel energetic or fatigued. No opponent regulates your speed; *you* do that. In games like tennis or handball you are at your opponent's mercy, as not a few tragic incidents involving individuals too proud to quit have demonstrated.

And here is the clincher! *Tests show that "most active" men have no advantage over "moderately active" men in the heart attack sweepstakes.* So your hard-driving, tennis-playing friend benefits no more than you and sometimes assumes some risk besides.

"I KNOW A FELLOW...."

Many people are ingenious in finding excuses for avoiding exercise. The overeater comforts himself with the familiar story of the person who never walked except to the dinner table and who nevertheless lived to a ripe old age.

Then there was the fellow who exercised every day, walked endlessly, ate wisely and dropped dead of a heart attack at the age of 40.

These tales may ease the conscience of the slothful, but they do not change the picture. The fact remains that if you exercise you have a much better chance of escaping a heart attack than your

17

sedentary friend has. And an even better chance of living if you do have a heart attack. We repeat this because it represents a situation that we must face honestly for our own benefit. The statistics should outweigh a whole battalion of exceptions you may have heard about. Remember—you may not be one of the lucky ones who disregards all health rules and gets away with it.

THE HOSPITAL WALK

Doctors are so sure of the benefits of exercise that they have even introduced it into the hospital room. After an operation they get a patient to his feet at the first possible moment. Deaths from embolism—sudden blood-vessel blockage—have dropped almost to the vanishing point since we started people walking after their operations. But don't delay *your* walking until that stage.

KNOWING IS NOT ENOUGH

To be aware that walking is good for you adds to your knowledge but not to your health. You must *do* something about it. The sad truth is that even after years of education and information programs by life insurance companies, medical associations, individual doctors and the Life Extension Institute, the President's Council on Physical Fitness can still report that "relatively few Americans get the regular, planned exercise which is basic to fitness in advanced societies."

As the Council points out: "The ordinary tasks of daily living no longer provide enough vigorous exercise to develop and maintain good muscle tone or cardiovascular and respiratory fitness."

2/The Perfect Exercise

Walking is an amazingly inclusive exercise—one that without the disadvantages of other exercises, helps your entire system function better. Your metabolism (the rate at which you burn up calories for vital bodily processes) goes up and your blood pressure down; blood cholesterol and sugar levels tend to fall, and the oxygen content of your blood stream is raised. All of this favors the burning up of fat and may help keep the arteries clear and elastic.

Further, your overall circulation is stimulated, improving not only your physical condition but also your morale or outlook on life. You take on the trim look of health. In brief, there is nothing to fear and everything to gain by the mild exercise of walking—at any age.

WHEN?

This is where the mental hazard comes in. Just as the equipment exerciser and the gym-goer tend to backslide, it may be hard for you to acquire new habits. Perhaps you are a television addict who cannot tear yourself away from the tube, whatever the program. This is not unusual—many intelligent people seem mesmerized by

TV even though they freely acknowledge that much of what they see is not worth looking at.

When you do leave the house, usually late because television never stops, it is almost second nature for you to hail a taxi or get on a bus even when you have only ten blocks to go.

In spite of all this, your advantage as a prospective walker is great—you do not have to put on special clothes or seek out an appropriate route. All you have to do is plan. But unless you *do* plan your walking each day, *you will not walk*. Good intentions may provide paving for the nether regions but they have never improved anyone's circulation.

So keep in mind that walking is not something you can do on the basis of "when I have a chance I'll do it." *You have to do it every day*. You must realize that your body needs exercise every day just as it needs food. You cannot exercise only on weekends and satisfy your body's requirements any more than you can eat just on weekends and take care of your nutritional needs.

IT WORKS!

Here is a program that is working for many men and women: First, they *think* in terms of walking. Then they establish an objective. Most have found that they get a lot out of walking for 20 minutes, two or three times a day. Some walk part of the way to work, getting off a train or bus before their destination to do so.

At lunch time, they choose a restaurant a ten-minute walk away, and walk to it and back again to their office. At night time, they repeat their morning routine, once more putting in 20 minutes of walking.

In this way they get their exercise and avoid the Big City Blues that frequently afflicts those of us whose business or profession makes it impossible for us to live in more natural surroundings. The great cities have dehumanizing effects against which we must ever be on guard.

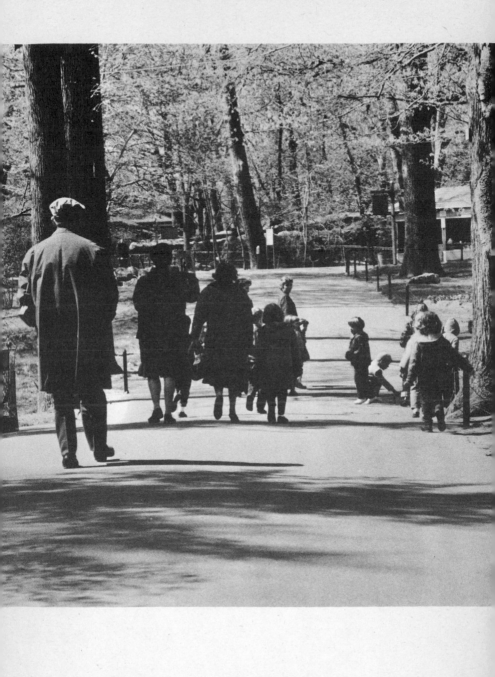

THE CREATIVE WALKING PROGRAM

There is a difference, of course, in the walking needs and capabilities of men and women. Children, too, are in a category of their own, but if they are permitted to exercise their natural vigor without coddling or over-protectiveness they will ordinarily get all the walking they require.

The President's Council on Physical Fitness and Sports has designated walking speeds as "slow," "moderate" and "fast." Although the rate which the Council deems "moderate" seems somewhat better than that to us, the Council chart should be helpful to men who want some guide to walking speed. We do not recommend the Council's "fast" pace of four and a half miles an hour except for brief intervals and for men in excellent physical condition.

Time for Various Distances

Distance	Time (Minutes : Seconds)		
	Slow Walk (3 mph)	Moderate Walk (4 mph)	Fast Walk (4.5 mph)
55 Yds.	:38	:28	:25
110 Yds.	1:15	:56	:50
220 Yds.	2:30	1:52	1:40
440 Yds.	5:00	3:45	3:20
880 Yds.	10:00	7:30	6:40
1 Mile	20:00	15:00	13:20

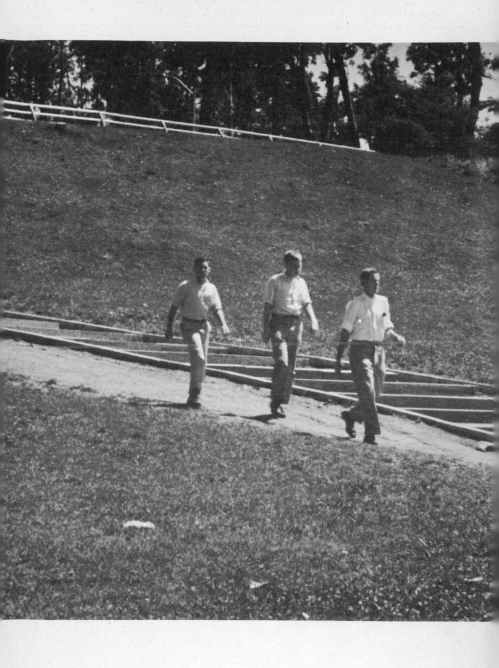

Plan A—FOR MEN

Accepting the Council's rating of walking speed, except for the "fast" pace, the following program is recommended for men who have not been exercising regularly but who do not feel that they are so far gone that they need the personal attention of a doctor or therapist. The key to progress is *every day*. When you start a walking program and then neglect it for a while, it is as if you had halted in the middle of climbing a mountain and slipped back to the bottom. Then you have to start the climb all over again.

Week 1

During this week, try to keep to level ground. Stay within the recommended distances even though you may feel you can do more.

Day 1	Walk 1 mile	slow
Day 2	Repeat Day 1	
Day 3	Walk 1½ miles	slow
Day 4	Repeat Day 3	
Day 5	Walk 2 miles	slow
Day 6	Repeat Day 5	
Day 7	Walk 2½ miles	slow

Week 2

Level ground walking is also specified for the second week. Try not to skip a day here and there with the thought of walking twice as far the next day. For best results, walking must be a habit.

Day 1	Walk 2½ miles	slow
Day 2	Repeat Day 1	
Day 3	Walk 3 miles	slow
Day 4	Repeat Day 3	
Day 5	Walk 3½ miles	slow
Day 6	Repeat Day 5	
Day 7	Walk 4 miles	slow

Week 3

By this week you should be over any initial muscle soreness and should be able to take longer distances. Short breaks are permissible—even advisable. There are no fixed rules, but the Army's five minutes an hour may be a guide. Again, do not go faster than the Council's "slow" pace of three miles an hour.

Day 1	Walk 4 miles	slow
Day 2	Repeat Day 1	
Day 3	Walk 4½ miles	slow
Day 4	Repeat Day 3	
Day 5	Walk 5 miles	slow
Day 6	Repeat Day 5	
Day 7	Walk 5½ miles	slow

Week 4

Your body should now be fit to accept more vigorous exercise in the form of the Council's "moderate" speed of four miles per hour. But cut down somewhat on distance at this speed.

Day 1	Walk 3 miles	moderate
Day 2	Repeat Day 1	
Day 3	Walk 3½ miles	moderate
Day 4	Repeat Day 3	
Day 5	Walk 4 miles	moderate
Day 6	Repeat Day 5	
Day 7	Walk 4½ miles	moderate

Week 5

In order to harden muscles and develop stamina, repeat the Week 4 schedule, except that you might try to find hillier country. Some uphill walking should give you the endurance for undertaking the more strenuous exercise that is scheduled at this point. When you repeat weeks according to instructions, do not start with the longest

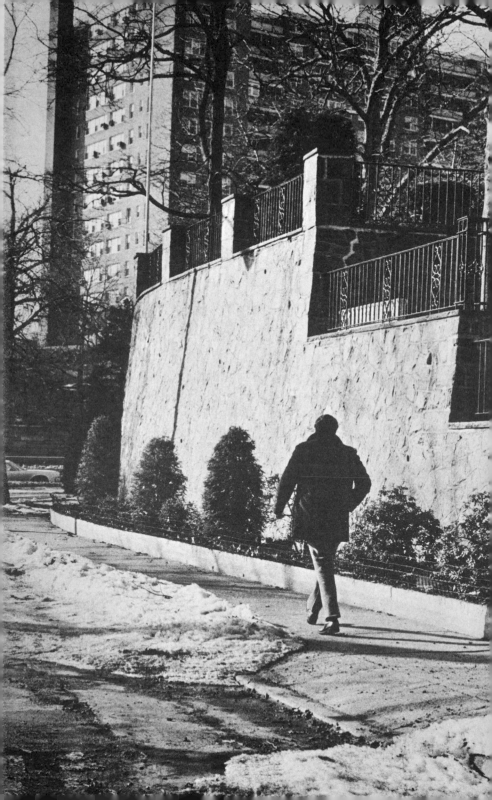

day's walk that was accomplished, but go back to the shorter distance—that is, the distance covered in Day 1 of the preceding week. This may seem like a retrogression, but in reality it serves to consolidate the gains you have made at the same time it prevents over-exertion.

Week 6

Since you are now half-way through your second month of creative walking, you should be able to handle the following program. However, if you find you are exceeding your strength or are dubious about the state of your health, it would be wise to see a doctor before going further. The chances are that he will be pleased at your condition, but if he does detect evidence of strain you may be wise to go back to the shorter distance and slower pace of Weeks 1 and 2 until you feel up to going ahead.

Day 1	Walk 5 miles	moderate
Day 2	Repeat Day 1	
Day 3	Walk 5½ miles	moderate
Day 4	Repeat Day 3	
Day 5	Walk 6 miles	moderate
Day 6	Repeat Day 5	
Day 7	Walk 6½ miles	moderate

Week 7

Repeat Week 6, keeping in mind the caution given in Week 5 about going back to the shorter distance in Day 1 of the preceding week as you commence the repetition.

Week 8

This time you increase your distance once again, but without increasing your rate of speed.

Day 1	Walk 6 miles	moderate
Day 2	Repeat Day 1	

Day 3	Walk $6\frac{1}{2}$ miles	moderate
Day 4	Repeat Day 3	
Day 5	Walk 7 miles	moderate
Day 6	Repeat Day 5	
Day 7	Walk $7\frac{1}{2}$ miles	moderate

Week 9

You should now be in condition to undertake longer walks, perhaps hikes in the countryside up to ten miles or more on all kinds of terrain. A Saturday or Sunday are the most suitable days, of course, in the case of an employed person.

Day 1	Walk 8 miles	moderate
Day 2	Repeat Day 1	
Day 3	Walk $8\frac{1}{2}$ miles	moderate
Day 4	Repeat Day 3	
Day 5	Walk 9 miles	moderate
Day 6	Repeat Day 5	
Day 7	Walk up to 10 miles	moderate

Week 10

The schedule for this week is suitable for a man on vacation or one who can take time off from his occupation. If you can manage a long walking trip in the country, you will reap the reward of your adherence to the program. You will find yourself able to walk long distances—up to 15 or 20 miles—with keen pleasure and with increasing benefit to your health.

After this tenth week, you should have developed the habit of walking and will probably find that you will *want* to get out for long walks on every possible occasion. Walking will have become a pleasure and not a duty.

When you go back to your city job, you may no longer have

28

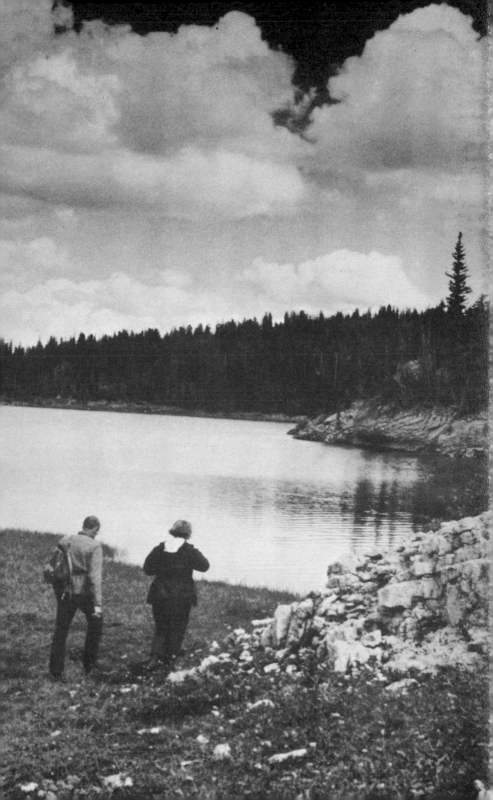

the time for seven or eight mile walks a day. If you are in good physical condition, as you should be after the amount of walking you have done, you may want to experiment with the Council's

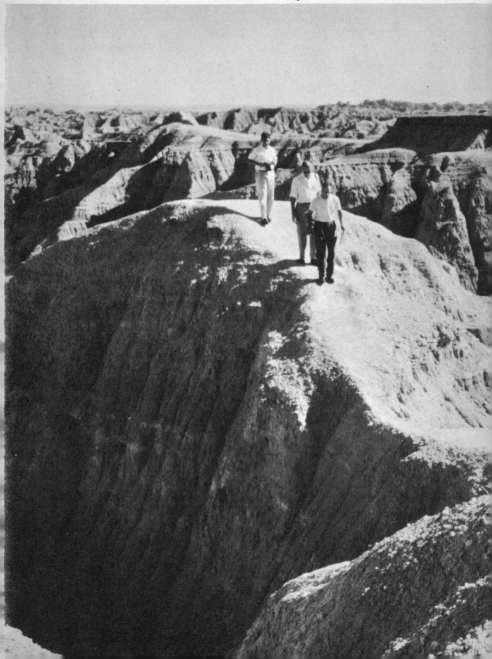

"fast" rate of four and a half miles an hour. But we believe you will find the "slow" or "moderate" rate more pleasurable and in the end more beneficial.

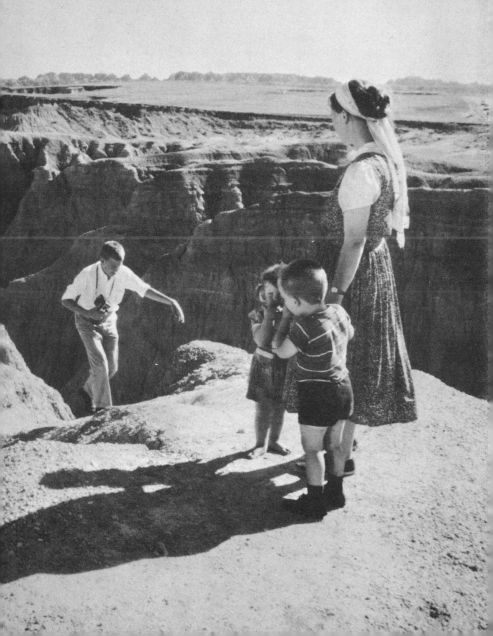

Plan B—FOR WOMEN

Most women would have trouble keeping up with the walking plan outlined for men. However, they should certainly try to follow a regular schedule like the one that will be suggested. Women need exercise as much as men do. Although their death rate from heart disease is not as high as that of men, women frequently suffer from unhappiness or depression as they take on weight and realize that they have lost some of their attractiveness. As crash diets and passive exercise plans prove worthless, they tend to lose faith in their ability to stay with any regular exercise program.

The fact is that the average housewife often believes firmly that she does enough exercise around the house without needing additional exercise, and she wonders why she does not lose weight. However, she has a built-in hazard—proximity to food throughout the day. If a hidden camera photographed every visit some women make to their refrigerators, the result would truly be an epicurean epic. A lot of this eating is done absent-mindedly, and at the end of the day the woman may say, quite honestly, that she has eaten very little. Then, one day, she looks in a full-length mirror and gasps in dismay. The Committee on Exercise and Physical Fitness of the American Medical Association explains why:

"One physician who has studied the problems of obesity in great detail has said that a woman would need to eat an average of only 96 calories a day more than she expends to gain 50 pounds from the time of her marriage to the arrival of her third child five years later. Had she added only 25 minutes of brisk walking to her daily activities, this weight gain would have been prevented."

In this case, the woman might have remained at her former weight by walking to the neighborhood grocery every day, instead of using the car.

The working woman, especially the one who works in an office, has a somewhat different problem. She does not have food con-

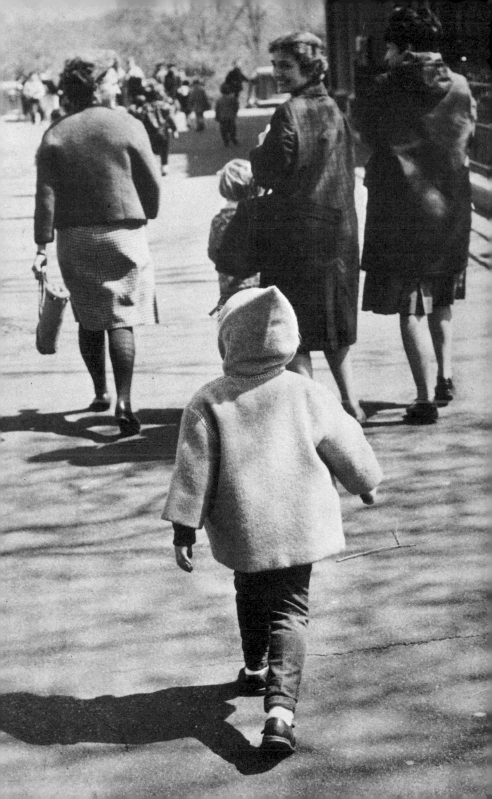

veniently close (except for the coffee-break cart) but she can easily fall into the habit of sitting most of the day. If she would make a deliberate effort to walk or climb stairs at every possible opportunity, she would avoid the middle-aged spread that makes so many working women unhappy.

Woman's physical makeup differs from that of man (remember the Frenchman who said "Vive le difference). This has to be taken into account when drawing up a walking program for her. Obviously, she is not as strong as a man; her bones are smaller and lighter and she is, over-all, less muscular. Moreover, since she is not usually as tall as a man, her stride is apt to be shorter. Finally, the structure of her pelvis differs from that of a male, resulting in greater pelvic rotation as she walks. This can be a source of some additional fatigue over the course of a lengthy walk.

Largely because of this, and because of psychological factors tied to the concept of femininity, we do not advise that a woman should ordinarily try to go beyond the pace that the President's Council designates as "slow"—that is, three miles an hour. But if a woman finds she can get up to three and a half miles an hour comfortably— perhaps in rural surroundings she need not feel inhibited about doing so. However, our plan calls for the slower pace, and the plan covers a period of nine weeks instead of the ten weeks of the man's program. At the end of the nine-week period, the woman walker should have settled comfortably into a routine that she can stay with indefinitely.

Week 1

As in the man's program, do not attempt rough or hilly country walking this first week. And make haste slowly.

Day 1	Walk 880 yds. ($\frac{1}{2}$ mile)	slow
Day 2	Repeat Day 1	
Day 3	Walk 1760 yds. (1 mile)	slow
Day 4	Repeat Day 3	
Day 5	Walk $1\frac{1}{2}$ miles	slow
Day 6	Repeat Day 5	
Day 7	Walk 2 miles	slow

34

Week 2

If you feel your muscles tightening up or if you feel extraordinarily tired, do not force yourself beyond your strength. You may decide that you do not want to tackle the Week 2 schedule yet, in which case you can repeat the Week 1 routine before going on to Week 2.

Day 1	Walk 2 miles	slow
Day 2	Repeat Day 1	
Day 3	Walk 2½ miles	slow
Day 4	Repeat Day 3	
Day 5	Walk 3 miles	slow
Day 6	Repeat Day 5	
Day 7	Walk 3½ miles	slow

Week 3

You may feel the need for breaks during your walks, so do not hesitate to take time out. The object of the plan is not to provide a punishing routine but to build up unused muscles gradually. Even if you feel vigorous, it will be better for you to repeat Week 2 at this point, starting with the shortest distance walked during that week.

Week 4

In the cause of moderation, which should be your watchword, you should observe a slight cutback in distance this week. You will benefit later on by building up your endurance slowly.

Day 1	Walk 1½ miles	slow
Day 2	Repeat Day 1	
Day 3	Walk 2 miles	slow
Day 4	Repeat Day 3	
Day 5	Walk 2½ miles	slow
Day 6	Repeat Day 5	
Day 7	Walk 3 miles	slow

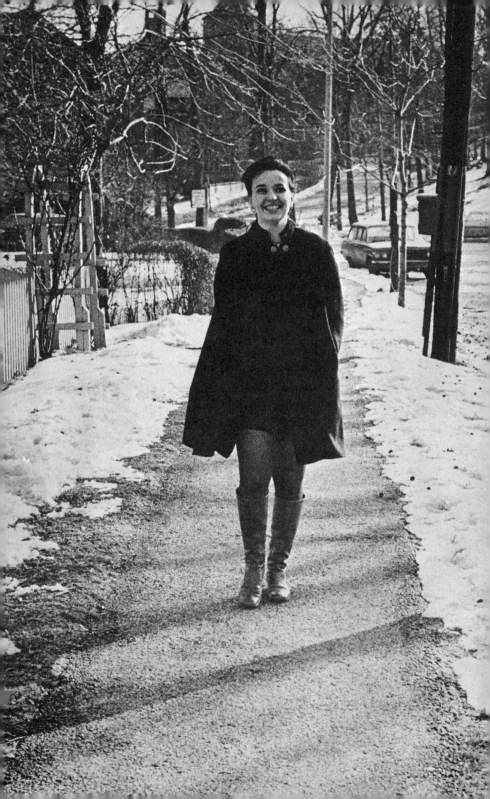

Week 5

Repeat Week 4. At this point you should be able to feel that your body is responding more easily to the demands you are putting on it.

Week 6

This is a good time to drop in on your doctor and have him check you. If you have been over-enthusiastic about your walking he may put in a word of caution, but the chances are that he will be highly pleased with your progress.

Day 1	Walk $2\frac{1}{2}$ miles	slow
Day 2	Repeat Day 1	
Day 3	Walk 3 miles	slow
Day 4	Repeat Day 3	
Day 5	Walk $3\frac{1}{2}$ miles	slow
Day 6	Repeat Day 5	
Day 7	Walk 4 miles	slow

Week 7

Repeat Week 6.

Week 8

Day 1	Walk $4\frac{1}{2}$ miles	slow
Day 2	Repeat Day 1	
Day 3	Walk 5 miles	slow
Day 4	Repeat Day 3	
Day 5	Walk $5\frac{1}{2}$ miles	slow
Day 6	Repeat Day 5	
Day 7	Walk 6 miles	slow

Week 9

This is the last week of your schedule. If it is possible, try to get out into the countryside for as long a walk as you find comfortable. It is quite possible that you may discover you can walk 10 miles or more without excessive fatigue. In the following weeks, try to continue the walking habit you have acquired. It will pay large dividends in better health and higher spirits.

FOR CHILDREN AND YOUNG PEOPLE

Regular walking, of course, is not only for those who feel the onset of middle age. It is important for every one. One of the so-called "advances" that is really retrogression is door-to-door bus service for school children. We do not know as yet what the effects of this practice are and we probably will not know for another twenty years. Some day, however, the present younger generation may awaken to the fact that, as a group, they are more prone to heart attacks than their forebears.

THE 4-F GENERATION

There is already some evidence of this from army draft examinations. There is a most disturbing lack of fitness among young men of an age that should see them at the peak of physical perfection. One draft board on Long Island in New York recently sent 100 young men to be examined for induction and 90 of them were rejected for physical and mental defects! As football coach Lynn Waldorf rightly told the American Academy of General Practice, "If our youths don't walk more, they'll wither."

MENTAL GIANTS—PHYSICAL PYGMIES

In recent years, colleges have been overemphasizing mental activity at the expense of physical exercise. Several years ago, Yale added its honored name to the long list of American colleges that have dropped compulsory gym. In Valhalla, those great if fictional Yalies, Frank and Dick Merriwell, must be burning the "Y"s they won on many an athletic battlefield. The old Greek concept of a sound mind in a sound body has been discarded. This lack of emphasis on physical well-being is extremely unfortunate. To a

38

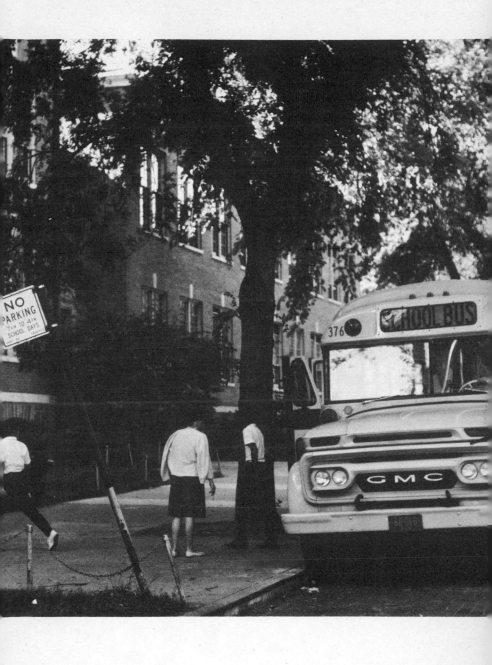

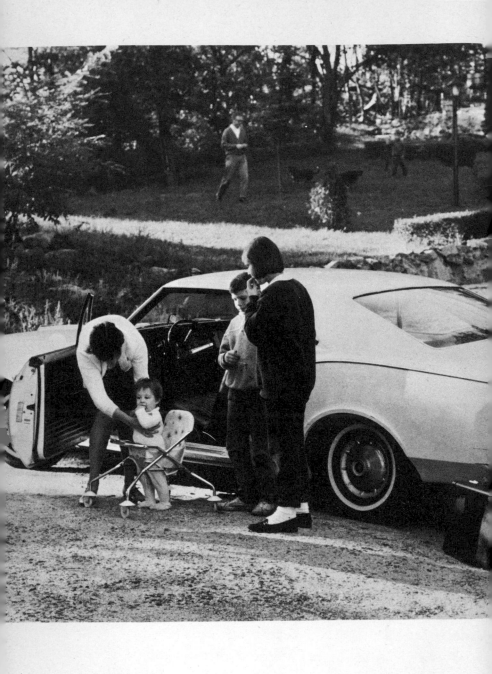

degree, it may be responsible for the emotional disturbances that so many college clinics report among their students, for mental health is often related to physical fitness. The individual who takes pride in his body is less likely to turn inward and brood on his problems.

We do not mean to disparage the work of psychiatrists—they are indispensable in our modern society—but in many cases of emotional "illness" that we have seen, we have felt that physical exercise and the glow of well-being it produces would be the best medicine.

TOO MUCH PROSPERITY?

We hear a great deal about deprivation and there is no doubt that there is a shameful amount of it in our country. But there is a corresponding amount of over-indulgence today, leading to the usual consequences of excess. The over-eating and over-drinking are one aspect of the affluent society. The 17- and 18-year-olds who drive their own cars are another. Perhaps this latter group are most to be pitied. Obviously, they get certain satisfactions out of their expensive automobiles. Yet they miss the exultation that comes from a long walk in the country, the stimulation of a walk through the city, developing their powers of observation and acquiring new insights.

The term "poor little rich boy" has long been out of fashion, but it still has validity. Witness the discontented generation, many of whose members are brighter than their predecessors and yet have lost touch with reality almost completely. Doctors see these young people when they become too ill to function even marginally, and they cannot help thinking that some wholesome exercise might have contributed to a more satisfactory way of life.

Perhaps it is time for the whole truth to be told about how the mental hospitals, state and private alike, are filling up with the boys and girls who sought *their* satisfaction in hallucinatory drugs after normal living had lost its meaning for them. The picture is a tragic one—far more tragic than most Americans realize. This damnable "mind expansion" philosophy, unless overcome, and speedily, can blast more of our youth than has the war in Viet Nam.

A normal teen-ager or boy or girl in the early 20's should certainly be able to keep up or go beyond the walking plans for men and women. If nothing else, adherence to the schedules will encourage the formation of life-long habits that can be infinitely rewarding.

For younger children, of course, the pediatrician is the best judge of how the child's feet can best grow normally. He can also advise on the nature and quantity of exercise the child should get. In most cases, his decision will be the more the better.

AFTER EATING?

For anyone—man, woman, or child—on the preceding program there is no harm in walking after eating. This is only unwise when there is some evidence of coronary insufficiency, and when chest pain is noted when walking after eating.

At the Life Extension Institute, men often tell us that they never have a chest pain except when they are walking to the train in the morning, after breakfast. Obviously, what happens is that they are in a hurry and walk rapidly. As a result, their coronary insufficiency causes anginal pain. The effort to digest food along with the effort of walking are a little more than the coronary circulation can comfortably handle. (It has been noted that commuters in the Greater New York area, especially on the Long Island and Penn Central railroads, are subject to special stresses which may have adverse physical effects.)

THEY WALK THEIR WAY TO HEALTH

It is the very people who experience some slight discomfort on exercising who *need* to walk. By doing so they improve their circulation, and many of them find after a while that they no longer have the alarming symptoms. It is by no means unusual to see a man who used to have to stop for a rest after walking a few blocks step out confidently for a brisk hike after a few months of regular mild exercise.

GET UP AND GLOW

You can experience that glow by going for a brisk walk. If you feel warmed up after 15 minutes of walking you will *know* you are on the right track. You will feel you have done something; possibly you will be perspiring slightly even in cool weather. These are the signs that you are throwing enough of a load on the heart for it to respond as it must to begin developing the supplemental circulation that is the goal.

Regular walking is the keynote of this program, so as a result we recommend that you keep a progress chart. The chart will also afford you enjoyment as you look back and measure your progress. Be sure to fill out the chart *each day* as soon as you return from your walk. Don't delay—as soon as you return from your walk. Keep the chart as follows:

1) Each day enter the walking schedule completed as 1-1, 1-2, 1-3, etc., meaning that you have completed the first day of the first week, the second day of the first week, and so forth.

2) Mark an "0" in the square if you completely miss a day.

3) Mark 5, 7½, or any number that approximates the distance in miles done hiking.

As you proceed, you may wish to keep a weight record as well.

PROGRESS CHART

Days of the Month	MONTHS											
	Jan	Feb	Mar	Apr	May	June	July	Aug	Sept	Oct	Nov	Dec
1												
2												
3												
4												
5												
6												
7												
8												
9												
10												
11												
12												
13												
14												
15												
16												
17												
18												
19												
20												
21												
22												
23												
24												
25												
26												
27												
28												
29												
30												
31												
TOTAL												

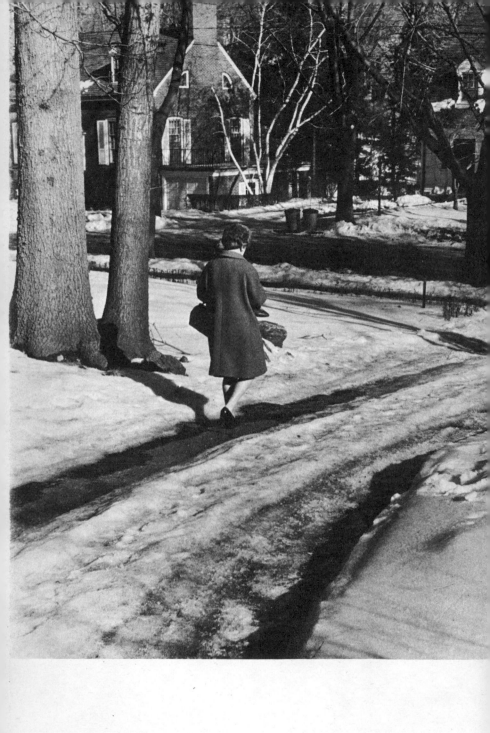

3/Old and Active

Whenever doctors see a person of advanced age who retains a zest for living, they generally find that he is physically active. There is something about sitting hour after hour that produces not only physical listlessness but an emotional torpor that is a kind of waiting for death. Former President Harry Truman more than once said about his morning walks, as youthful reporters tried to keep pace with him, "I believe it will make me live longer."

Mr. Truman has plenty of basis for his belief. We see so many people in their eighties and even in their nineties who have been good walkers all their lives. They developed the habit in a simpler age before the combustion engine took over our civilization. Dr. Paul Dudley White, the famous cardiologist, has told of one of his patients, aged 102, whom he advised to keep on walking just as he had always done. The man lived to be 107.

Of course, very few of those who walk regularly can expect to duplicate the feat of Dr. White's patient. There are too many factors involved in longevity—including heredity—for any one of them to be controlling. Nevertheless, we do know that the best way to keep old people from becoming invalided is to keep them active. And for these older folks—as well as for every one else—walking is the

47

best exercise. As Dr. White says: "A five-mile walk is better for the health of anyone not already too ill to walk than all the medicine and philosophy in the world."

Mind you, you may not be able to *reverse* the course of degenerative disease by walking. But you *frequently can slow further impairment.*

NOTHING BETTER

It is not easy to convince some people that walking *is* the best exercise. They think there must be a quicker, more modern way. And, as their gym memberships run out unused and their exercising equipment remains untouched, they deprive themselves of the walking that can do so much for their present and future health. The human body has not changed so much as to require ingenious new exercises. The oldest exercise is still the best.

4/Walking and Weight

One of the helpful aspects of walking is that it makes you health-minded. Thus, it is an important part of any weight-reducing routine. Even if you do not change your diet, an hour's walk a day will produce a loss of a pound a month. This does not sound like a great deal—but as you keep walking, more pounds come off. And they do not go right back on again, as happens when a person undertakes violent exercise and then relapses into his former sloth. But beyond this, once you have embarked on a walking program, you will undoubtedly find that you will want to be wiser about the food you eat. Indirectly, therefore, your walking will lead you into better practices in other health areas.

PROTECTING THEIR INVESTMENT

This kind of by-product—the encouragement of other sensible life programs—is well known to the vendors of weight-reducing devices that call for little or no effort on the part of the user. Once the individual has invested a substantial sum of money in such equipment, he tends to cut down on his food consumption in order to get the best results. Consequently, many men and women who

49

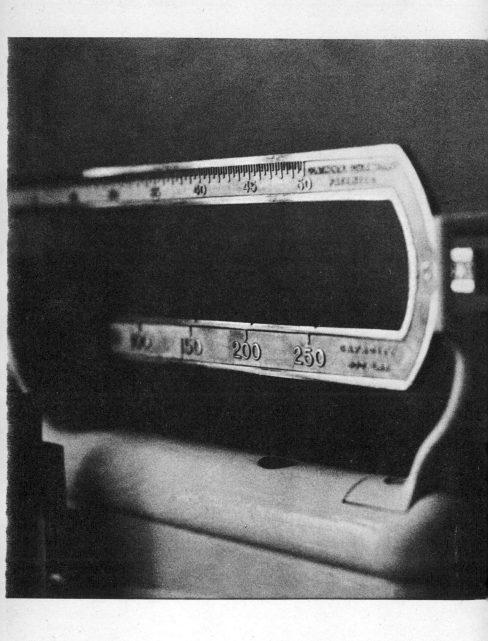

attribute their weight loss and better health to the use of one of the massage or passive exercise machines should credit their reduced diet instead.

WALKING YOUR STOMACH AWAY

There are other benefits from walking beyond those which come from the building up of collateral heart circulation. By stimulating the body's metabolism—the rate at which energy is made available to your body—walking aids weight loss. It strengthens the abdominal muscles and helps melt away the flabby flesh which is not only unsightly but which is so discouraging to those who want to look better but don't know how. Lack of morale, with its attendant pessimism, can be more damaging to health than some germs we know about.

START SLOW—THEN FULL SPEED AHEAD

Keep in mind that even with such a mild exercise as walking, some reasonable caution should be observed. If you haven't been doing any walking to speak of, begin your walking program by degrees. Start doing ten minutes at a slow pace and then gradually work up to a half hour at a brisk pace twice a day. Three or three-and-a-half miles an hour—a little more than an average city block a minute—is good speed. Then, if you feel comfortable and want to do more, by all means go ahead. And don't worry about any slight muscle aches—they will disappear as you get into shape.

RED LIGHT ROUTINE

If you walk in the city, you may find yourself stopped by a traffic light. If you are, follow this routine: Stand tall, tuck in your abdomen, squeeze your buttocks together, and take a deep breath or two. You will be improving your carriage as you avoid risking sudden death by crossing against the light.

51

5/Middle-Aged for Life!

Walking has one big advantage over jogging, aside from the fact that it is so much more convenient and requires no special clothes. For a person past the age of 50 who takes on a jogging program, the potential danger outweighs any benefit. Brisk walking is infinitely safer. It will not keep you young, mind you; inevitably the body changes with time. *But it can keep you middle-aged for life.* It lengthens the middle-aged plateau and keeps you from getting old *before* your time.

FIGHTING TENSION

One of the factors that makes a person old is worry and tension. Dr. White believes that walking is the best anti-tension procedure there is. If, for example, you can get out for a brisk walk after a trying business discussion, it will do you a lot more good than taking a tranquillizer or going to a bar.

AND IT'S FUN!

Above all—and this is what makes walking the universal exercise—most people get real pleasure out of it once they have given

52

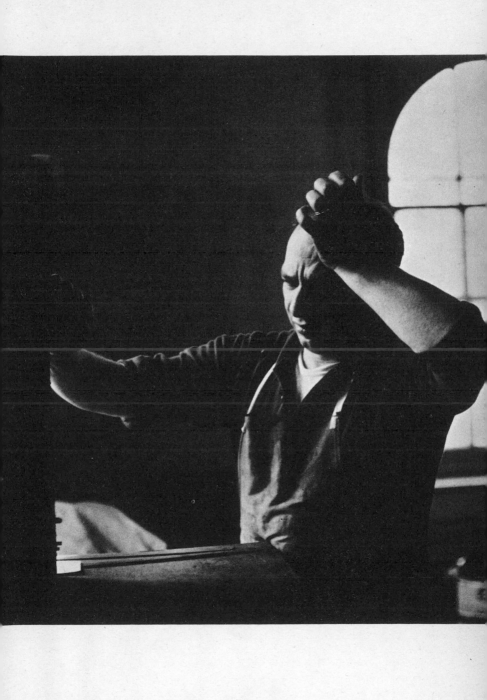

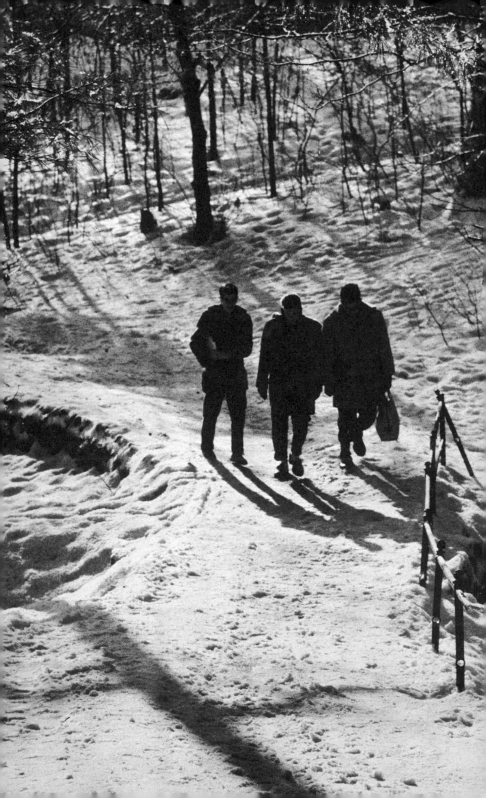

it a chance. Many get into the habit of walking two miles in the morning and two more at night. If they walk in the city, they develop the habit of observing happenings about them. There is one doctor from rural Virginia who likes to walk in New York City just to "watch the people." Country walks, of course, are rewarded by close contact with the beauties of nature. That is why walking, wherever it is done, is seldom boring.

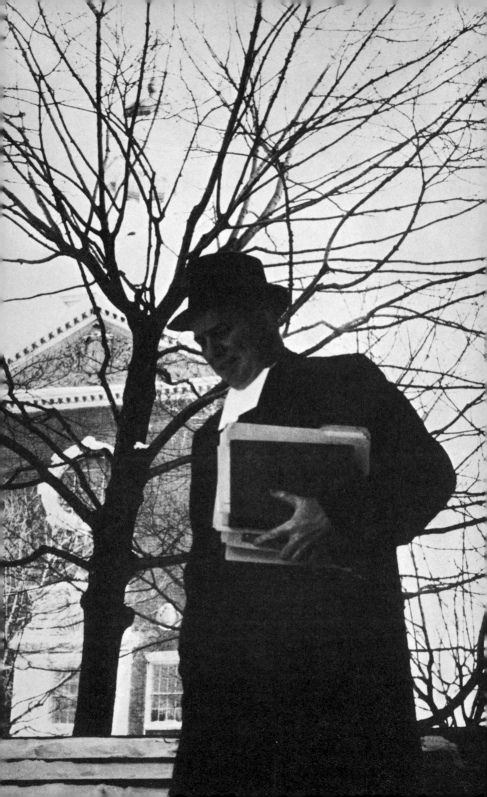

6/Walking and the Subconscious

A great many people, including both the man in the street and the greatest intellects of the day, have discovered benefits in walking that go far beyond those that pertain *directly* to health. Supreme Court Justice William O. Douglas has said that when he has a knotty legal case to consider, the best thing he can do is go for a walk. He has discovered over the years that at some time during the walk, or soon afterwards, the right answer will flash into his mind.

Judge Douglas' experience has been shared by thousands. Professional men—business men—all those who are confronted with problems that sometimes seem to defy solution, have learned that they can put their subconscious to work profitably by deliberately thrusting the vexing question out of their minds and going for a walk. Some have become so accustomed to find inspiration during a walk that they are never dismayed when they cannot come up with an answer quickly. They have confidence in this amazing thing that happens over and over again.

We are not sure why and how this comes about. But we know that it *does*. Apparently a reasonably lengthy walk by one's self stimulates the mind to fresh thinking and new insights. One prominent lawyer has said that an hour's walk frequently does him more good than a whole day spent in the law library. To borrow a thought from the psychologists, it may well be that the subconscious does its best work when you stop trying too hard.

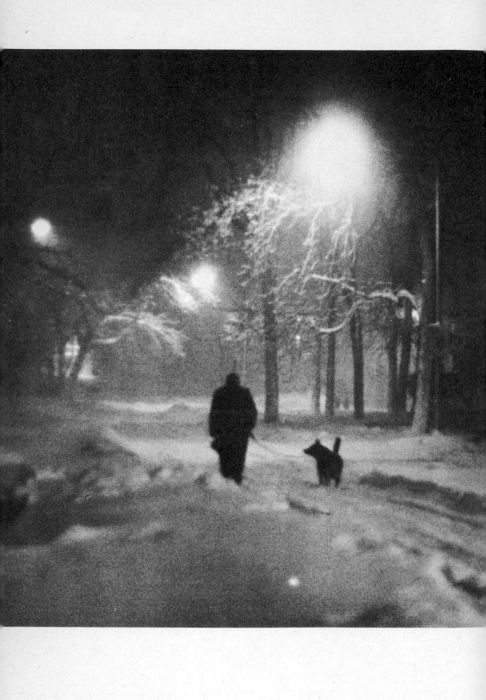

7/Walking and Your Moods

If you are annoyed or irritated, fed up with life, you can often get back on an even keel by taking a walk. Listen to the writer Donald Culross Peattie: "I have often started off on a walk in the state called mad—mad in the sense of sore-headed, or mad with tedium or confusion; I have set forth dull, null and even thoroughly discouraged. But I never came back in such a frame of mind, and I never met a human being whose humor was not the better for a walk."

THE INFLUENCE OF THE MIND

But what has Peattie's statement got to do with a person's health? A great deal. There is all about us today a tremendous amount of illness stemming from emotional factors; a person who cannot cope with the difficulties that life presents to all of us, sooner or later, in one form or another, will usually come up with a full-fledged set of psychosomatic ailments—illnesses that arise in the mind and affect the body. Anything that helps us deal more efficiently with our work or with any of the problems of living is all to the good. When so simple an exercise as walking can pay such dividends how unwise it is not to take advantage of it!

59

8/How to Walk

Shuffling along with your head down and your abdomen thrust forward is both unsightly and inefficient. Head up, stomach in, chest out, and an easy, comfortable, long stride with the toes pointed straight ahead are most likely to accomplish your purpose of physical and mental refreshment.

Walking is such a natural activity however that you do not have to memorize a set of rules and regulations, or keep a chart of your progress. Unless you are a born accountant who gets pleasure out of graphs and diagrams, you are better off without them. They can turn any pleasurable activity into a chore. Moreover, "evidences" of progress can be deceptive. You may do better on some days than on others, without any logical explanation. Sometimes physical progress is a matter of two steps forward and one step back.

Once you make sure you are wearing comfortable, well-fitting shoes, don't worry too much about "form." You will quickly find a way of walking that is best suited to you, even if it lacks something in grace. After all, you are not walking for applause or for points in a competition. You are walking for your life.

WALKING FOR SHEER PLEASURE

As you continue to make a habit out of walking, you will find yourself thinking less and less about the physical rewards. It is usually at this very point that the benefits really begin to mount up. In your enjoyment of the exercise, you will improve in health, spirits and mental alertness almost automatically. Weeks may pass without your stepping on a scale, measuring your waistline or trying to feel your pulse.

WALKING AWAY FEARS

This absorption in the pleasurable activity of walking is particularly helpful to the over-fearful, worrisome type of individual we call a hypochondriac. Unfortunately, we see more and more of these every year. People who are concerned about war, the nuclear bomb, and the other tremendous issues of the day about which they can do very little, tend to turn in upon themselves. Pretty soon they find all sorts of imaginary ailments.

If we can get these people to walk, the exercise not only distracts them from their "hang-ups," but it also gives them much-needed reassurance that they are actively doing something about their health. This can be more useful than the tranquillizers and pep up pills that Americans swallow by the billions each year. This craze for health in a bottle or a pill has made certain pharmaceutical companies immensely prosperous, with very little to show in the way of improved health for the customers.

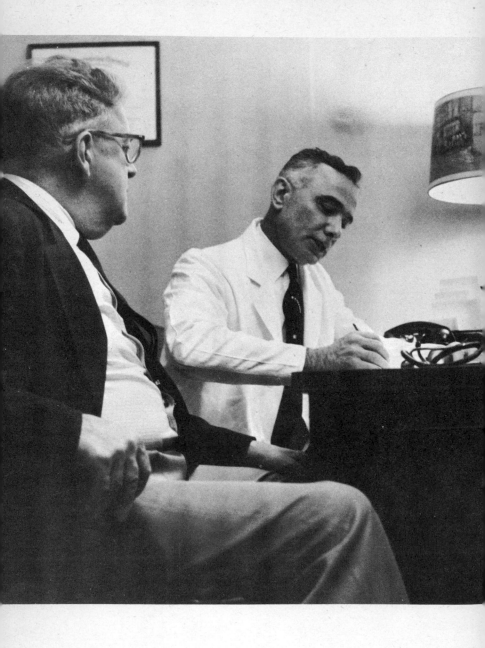

9/See the Doctor?

Because of the mildness of the exercise provided by walking, it is usually not necessary for you to get medical advice before you start unless you have reason to believe you have some physical ailment. This is another advantage you have over the person who goes in for jogging or one of the other more strenuous exercises. Too many of these people fail to get the necessary medical check-up before embarking on an ambitious program of exercise that may do them more harm than good. We have seen plenty of them who go at their exercises as if they were getting ready for the next Olympic Games.

RECRUITS TO THE RANKS

Many of these over-sold individuals eventually see the light and join the ranks of the walkers. Unfortunately, many delay switching because before they do so they must get over the feeling that the more you do of something and the harder you work at it the better off you are. But in exercising, the law of diminishing returns sets in rather quickly. Usually it begins to operate just about the time that the unfavorable effects of over-exertion become evident.

WHAT THE EXPERTS SAY

Because doctors have seen too many of the consequences of unreasonably vigorous exercise, some of them are "bearish" on the

63

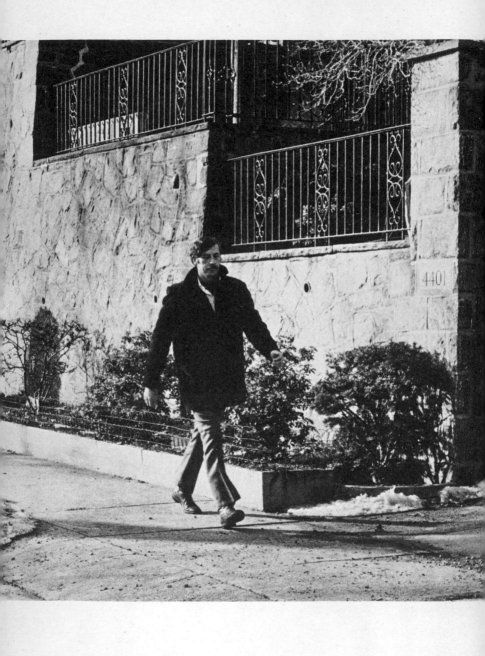

whole idea of exercise. But by and large most of them agree that walking combines excellent results with a minimum of risk.

Those who are still cautious about the possibility of strain in even so mild an exercise as walking should be reassured by a report by Dr. Dale Groom, professor of medicine and associate dean of the University of Oklahoma School of Medicine. "Most of us," Dr. Groom says, "brought up in our comfortable and sedentary civilizations, actually develop and use only a fraction of our potential cardiac reserve."

This potential is there, but one must reach for it wisely. Dr. Howard A. Rusk, the famous specialist in rehabilitation and also an outstanding author, in describing the physical feats of a Mexican Indian tribe, points out that they "have conditioned themselves through their whole life, in contrast to the uninformed joggers or would-be athletes who try to go the distance the first day."

Adds Dr. Rusk: "An example of this is a New York industrialist, now deceased, who was told by his doctor that what he needed was exercise and to go out and run around the reservoir in Central Park. At the end of the run, on his very first day, he collapsed with his first coronary occlusion."

"The greatest antidote for overexercise tragedies," Dr. Rusk concludes, "is common sense."

The American Heart Association agrees. "*Walking briskly*," it states, "*not just strolling, is the simplest and also one of the best forms of exercise.*"

The final word comes from the Metropolitan Life Insurance Company which is very much interested in keeping people alive, both for their own sakes and for the sake of the company's fine financial structure. "Exercise," the Metropolitan says, "does not have to be either laborious or time-consuming. One of the simplest ways is to walk when you do not absolutely have to ride. Walking is a fine way to keep yourself in good shape."

With such impressive backers, one can hope that some day walking will be accepted for the great medicine it is, even though it does not possess the glamor of better-publicized forms of exercise.

65

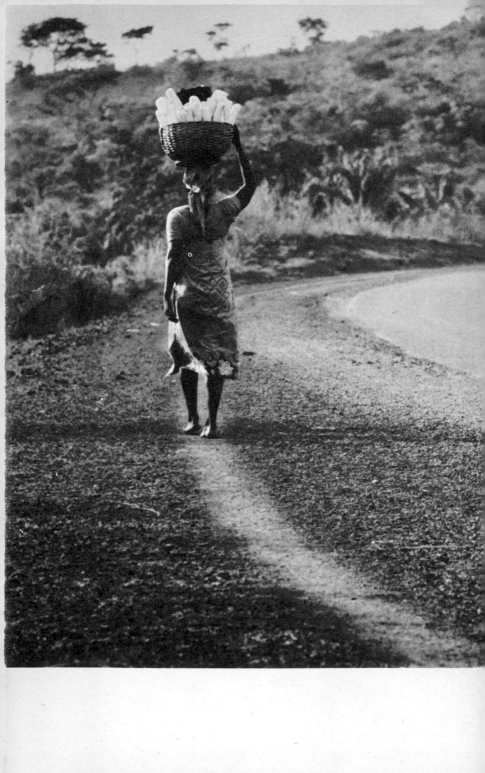

10/It Goes Way Back

If you do become a habitual walker, you will have a lot of tradition behind you—a million years of it in fact—and besides you will be carrying on as a higher primate should. John Napier, reader in anatomy at the Royal Free Hospital School of Medicine of the University of London, makes this interesting comment in *Scientific American*: "The fact that man has used this form of locomotion (walking) for more than a million years has only recently been demonstrated by fossil evidence. The antiquity of this human trait is particularly noteworthy because walking with a striding gait is probably the most significant of the many evolved capacities that separate men from more primitive hominids."

It only remains to be said that when our astronauts arrived on the moon they did not jog, they did not bicycle, they did not play handball—they walked!

The defense rests.

67

11/Walking and Well-Being

Because walking is not the whole of living (even if an important part of it), it is difficult to exclude from any discussion about it other aspects of sound health practice. Once you have begun to improve your overall condition by wise walking, you will find that various troublesome health problems tend to disappear. And even if they persist in some measure, you may gain something that is exceedingly important: a sense of well-being.

The enjoyment of life summed up in the phrase "a sense of well-being" is not usually dependent on one's circumstances in life or even on the presence or absence of difficulties. Another word for it is "zest," and that is precisely the feeling that so many seem to lack today. Even when they cannot identify any real troubles in their lives, they go about with an apathetic, dragged-out look that says very eloquently that they are just not having any fun.

When one considers the relative shortness of life, it seems a shame

68

to spend any part of it—much less a substantial portion—in what can only be described as a zombielike condition. Mind you, those who suffer from this kind of "soul sickness" would like nothing better than to be free of it. That is why they go from one "miracle pill" to another, never quite finding the right one. One nostrum may work for a while, not because of any intrinsic value but on the placebo, or sugar pill, principle. It works because the person *thinks* he is getting a potent medicine, not because he actually is. But before long the same old depression returns.

The tragic thing is that so many are suffering unnecessarily. If they would get the walking habit they might very quickly find that such a simple procedure as getting up out of their easy chairs and moving their legs vigorously for an hour would do wonders for their outlook on life.

Obviously, there are people who are so emotionally ill that more stringent measures are required. But this number is small in comparison with the vast majority who need only to be jolted out of their lethargy and indifference.

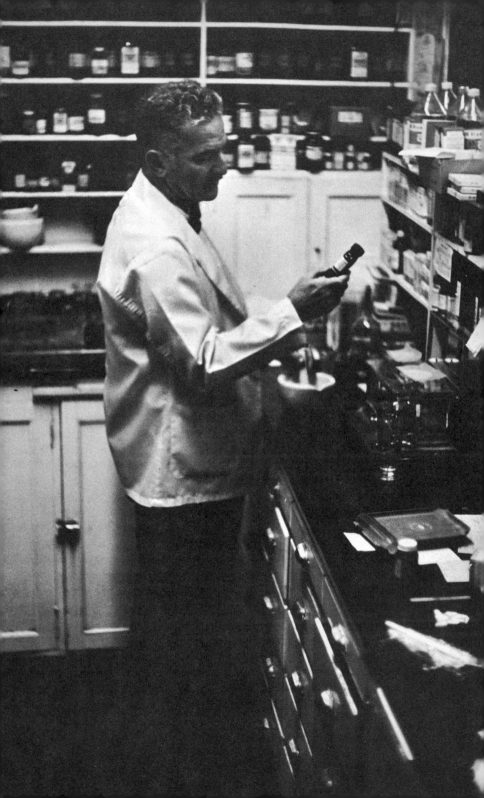

12/Walking and Sleep

One of the greatest enemies of the sense of well-being in this age is the inability to sleep. After a few sleepless nights, most people are not fit to be lived with. Ordinarily courteous and well-mannered individuals will snarl at the slightest provocation, much to the detriment of their family and social life. These people are greatly to be pitied, especially since the fatigue and tension they feel often prevent them from seeking a sane solution. We do not claim that walking by itself will cure insomnia, but as it relieves tension and induces moderate fatigue without stimulation, it can be an important part of a cure.

Unfortunately, many victims of insomnia turn to sleeping pills, some more potent than others. These aids to sleep can do more harm than good. The sleep they induce is frequently more like a drugged slumber than natural rest, and the cumulative effects of taking them can be both addictive and dangerous.

This is not the place to retell the many stories of sleeping pill addicts who found death in an overdose taken because they were too dazed to remember that they had already taken their pills. And for every one of these unfortunate fatalities, there are thousands of other men and women who depend on barbiturates for what is essentially an inferior kind of sleep, and who eventually need stronger and stronger doses until their health breaks down.

71

13/Walking and Overeating

Nearly everyone knows at least one compulsive eater who keeps "snacking" because he is unwittingly trying to make up for some lack in his life. If the glutton doesn't find a better way to work off his tensions, he is inviting a whole series of physical ailments—with a possible heart attack in the front rank.

At the risk of laboring the point, here again vigorous walking can help drain off the tension that often leads to overeating. And contrary to an old myth, this kind of *mild exercise* does not make one hungrier and thus lead to further eating. On the contrary, by helping create a new, vigorous approach to life it encourages wiser diet habits in the same way that it encourages so many other sound habits.

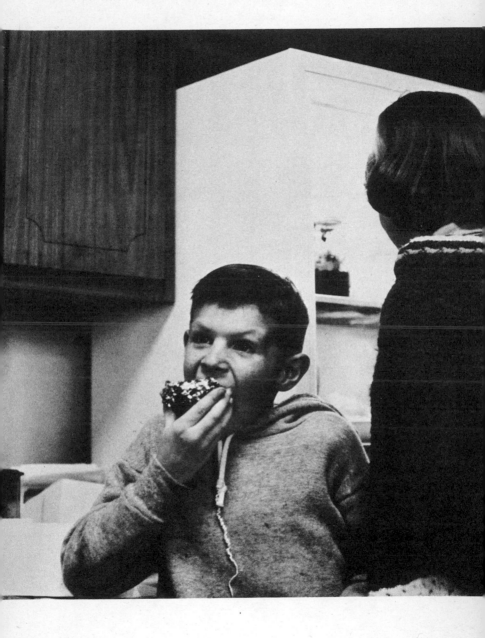

14/Walking and Alcohol

With the emphasis in recent years on drug addiction, we have been hearing less about over indulgence in alcohol. Nevertheless, alcoholism remains an enormous problem in our own country and indeed throughout the world. It would take a book by itself to record the toll of human wreckage and financial loss for which this disease—and it is a disease—has been responsible. Fully recognizing that we may appear to be putting forward walking as a universal panacea, we still feel strongly that vigorous walking can help with the psychological stresses that often lead to excessive drinking. We also believe that it can help give the compulsive drinker the perspective on himself and his relationship to those about him that he sorely needs.

To sum up, walking can help put him on the path to moderation. This is not as hopeless as many believe, as the large number of formerly heavy drinkers who have been "on the wagon" for years indicates.

15/Other Exercises?

Perhaps the impression has been given that you should forego every kind of exercise except walking. Of course, this has not been intended. If you enjoy bicycling, bowling or swimming, or if you are the rare individual who gets pleasure out of calisthenics—fine. If you are a golfer, certainly no one has to persuade you to get out on the course. However, you might try dispensing with the cart that moves you from hole to hole and let your feet provide the transportation.

But whatever kind of other exercise you do, don't stop walking! Over the long run you will find it is the most available, the least expensive and the most productive exercise there is.

In many parts of the country, the weather may not be suitable for walking for days at a time. There is nothing wrong with walking in the rain or snow, and in fact many people derive pleasure from it. But extremes of heat or cold may call for some caution in walking. Therefore, we are appending a five-minute program of

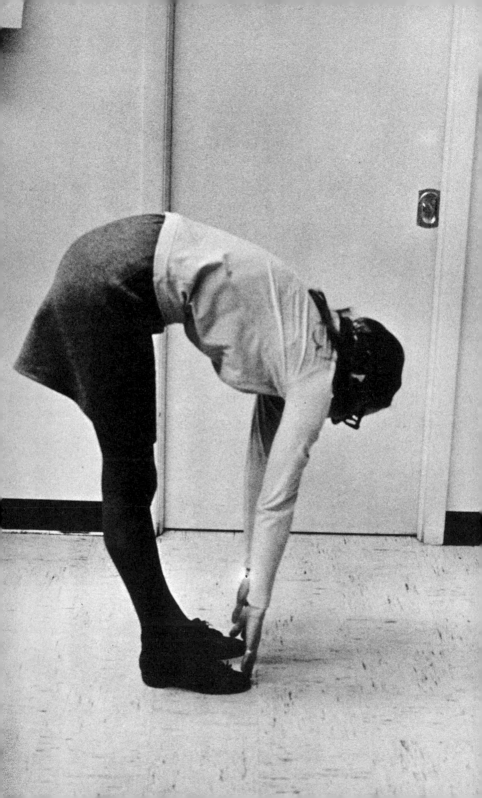

exercises that will help keep you in condition if you are obliged to cut down on your walking:

1. Stretch and Breathe

Extend your arms over your head; stand on your toes, stretch, and inhale. Then exhale and relax to normal standing position. *Repeat 12 times.*

2. Trunk Bending (forward)

Stand with your feet together, knees straight, hands on hips. Bend forward from the waist at right angles to the legs; keep the back flat and the chin extended. *Repeat 12 times.*

3. Trunk Bending (sideways)

Stand with your feet apart, hands over head. Bend slowly to the left as far as possible. Return to upright position. *Repeat 6 times to the left, 6 times to the right.*

4. Knee Bending

Stand with your feet slightly apart, hands on hips. Bend knees slowly; go down as far as possible without lifting heels from ground. Rise slowly to upright position. *Repeat 12 times.*

5. Bicycle

Lie on your back. Support back at waist with hands and bent elbows, carrying your weight between head and elbows as if you were trying to push your hips up to the ceiling. Now bend and extend your legs alternately, just as if you were riding a bicycle. *Repeat 20 times,* or until you feel *slightly tired.*

16/Fat—The Enemy

Since our goal in this book is to be practical and realistic, we must emphasize that you can walk and walk and walk, but if you insist on adhering to unwise eating habits, in the long run all your efforts will be either useless or only half successful. If one of your problems is obesity, the direction of your walk should be away from the table and the refrigerator.

The following is a useful weight chart that can give you some idea of what you should weigh:

Average Weights of Men

Graduated weights (indoor clothing and shoes) in pounds

Height**	Age: 30–39	40–49	50–59	60–69
5′0″	131	134	136	133
1″	134	137	139	136
2″	137	140	142	139
3″	141	144	145	142
4″	145	148	149	146
5″	149	152	153	150
6″	153	156	157	154

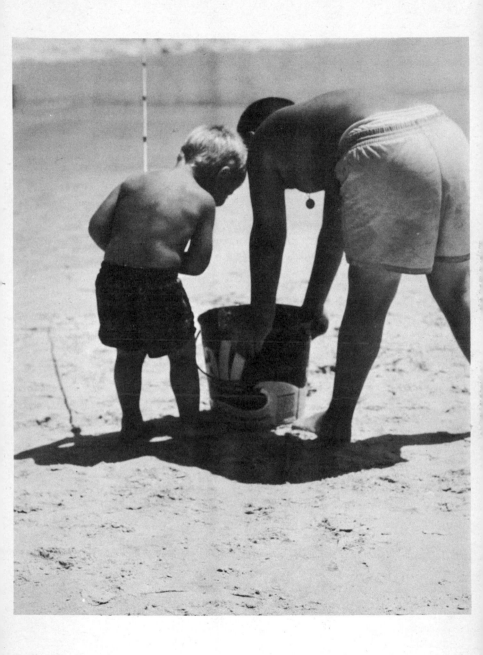

7"	157	161	162	159
8"	161	165	166	163
9"	165	169	170	168
10"	170	174	175	173
11"	174	178	180	178
6'0"	179	183	185	183
1"	183	187	189	188
1"	188	192	194	193
3"	193	197	199	198
4"	199	203	205	204

Average Weights of Women

Graduated weights (indoor clothing and shoes) in pounds

Height**	Age: 30–39	40–49	50–59	60–69
4'10"	115	122	125	127
11"	117	124	127	129
5'0"	120	127	130	131
1"	123	130	133	134
2"	126	133	136	137
3"	129	136	140	141
4"	132	140	144	145
5"	135	143	148	149
6"	139	147	152	153
7"	142	151	156	157
8"	146	155	160	161
9"	150	159	164	165
10"	154	164	169	*
11"	159	169	174	*
6'0"	164	174	180	*

*Average weights omitted in classes having too few cases.
**Men add one inch for shoes; women add two inches.

But even without the chart, there is an easy way of finding out if you are overweight.

1. Lie on your back. If your stomach is flat, you are not unduly fat. If it is higher than your chest, you may well be.

2. Standing up, pinch the flesh beneath your ribs between your index finger and thumb. If your fingers are more than an inch apart, start reducing.

PRACTICE WHAT THEY PREACH?

There is a vast difference between knowing what to do and doing it. That is why so many doctors, even though they are fully aware of the health rules, often violate them flagrantly. A doctor we know warns his patients against the consequences of lack of exercise, while the only exercise *he* gets consists of lifting a stethoscope and writing prescriptions. Some years ago, a physician who issued frequent statements on the dangers of being overweight on behalf of a large insurance company, was himself some 40 pounds overweight.

You cannot expect *your* doctor, therefore, always to set you a good example in health matters. (The fact is that a doctor's life averages five years shorter than that of the general population. Overwork and lack of exercise take their toll.) But you *can* follow his advice which will probably be much the same as that which you are reading in this book. If you do, you may within a reasonable time feel like one middle-aged man who, after years of "relaxation," began taking daily walks. Contrasting his previous lethargy with his new-found zest for living, he made this comment: "It's like having another sense."

Many other walkers have expressed much the same idea. After they begin walking regularly, their only regret is that they spent so many years "sitting around." "It's like those old ads about wasted time—the years that the locusts have eaten," one man said.

MAN AND THE MACHINE

It cannot be emphasized too strongly that the age of automation has begun to turn many people into servants of the machine. In the process they have gradually lost much of the independence of spirit and the personal initiative that our forefathers possessed. It

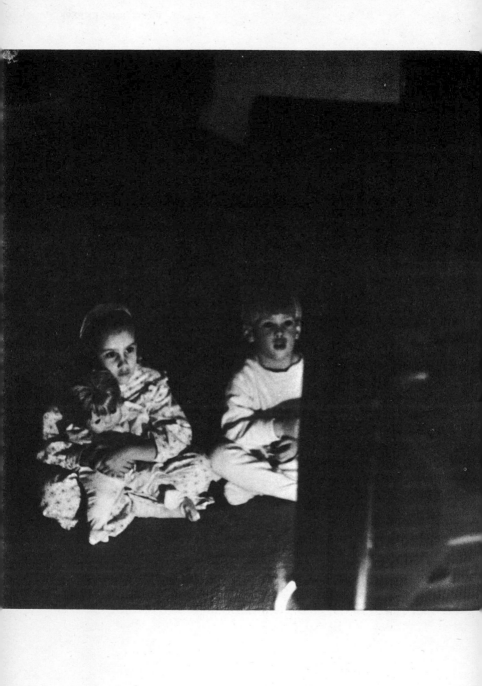

is not easy for such people to break long-standing habits and to rouse themselves, even when their lives are at stake.

It is somehow symptomatic of today's "standards" that remote control of television channel changing has become increasingly popular. Now you don't even have to move out of your easy chair or bed to switch from John Wayne to Ed Sullivan. You just push a button. The few feet to the television set have become too far to walk.

These very words—*Too Far To Walk*—became the title of a novel by a perceptive writer, John Hersey. Hersey describes how aimlessness and boredom make even a stroll to a nearby lecture hall too much for a young man. This is what we must struggle against—the pervasive hollowness that makes anything more strenuous than pushing a button an effort.

WHAT COUNTS

At the Life Extension Institute we have come to recognize that energy, vitality, *élan vital*—call it what you will—is the one most important attribute for success in life. In many cases, in fact, it makes up for the absence of great ability or talent. There are so few who can throw themselves whole-heartedly into a project that they are often prized above those who may be brainier or better informed. And one way of developing this kind of enthusiasm is by sound, sensible, non-destructive exercise. Those heroes of the detective stories who never move from their rooms and rely entirely on "deduction" from facts others bring to them, are creatures not of this world. No one sunk in such lassitude could possibly solve anything more difficult than two plus two.

THE MYSTERY

Consider how strange it is that one should have to force oneself to perform such an utterly natural act as walking. But we must reckon with the unfortunate tendency of the human species to emulate the two-toed sloth. Fortunately for man, the process of breathing is automatic or we would find thousands dying daily of

83

asphyxiation. When we see so many individuals flagrantly inviting trouble, we wonder whether the psychiatrists may not be right about the "death wish" they attribute to some of their patients. Authorities on Oriental and African cultures have described instances of individuals making up their minds to die and dying shortly afterwards. Are we moving in that direction?

17/Tired?

Every doctor in general practice knows the patient who complains he is always tired. Almost automatically, the doctor presumes that the fatigue does not arise out of overwork—quite the contrary. In the vast majority of cases, the man or woman has just gone slack for want of exercise. The muscles are without tone, the whole body droops in a kind of "sad sack" attitude that comes from prolonged inactivity.

Unfortunately, a person in such a situation usually believes it is impossible for him to do anything that requires even the minimum of effort. As a result, the degeneration of his physique continues until his body cannot resist illnesses that ordinarily would be of little consequence. The number of chronic invalids and semi-invalids in our country is an indication of how we have allowed ourselves to deteriorate.

If *you* feel tired all the time don't jump to the conclusion that you need one of the patent medicines recommended by one of the impressive-sounding pitchmen (usually in a white coat) who are heard endlessly on TV. You should, of course, have a doctor examine you to determine whether there is any organic reason for your lack of energy. Once this possibility is eliminated, try to remember

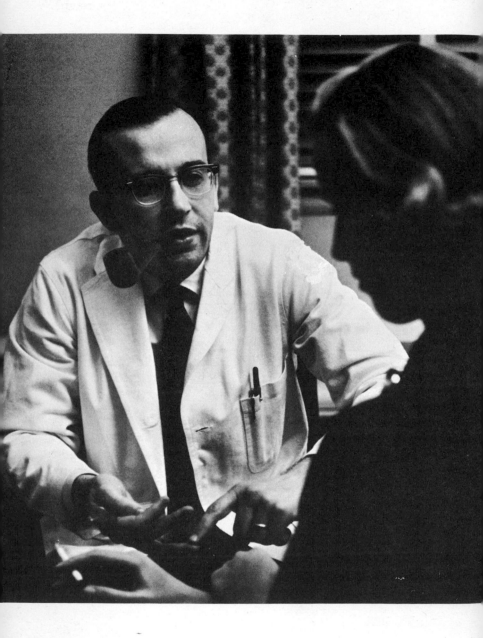

what a president of the American Medical Association said: "It begins to appear that exercise is the master conditioner for the healthy and the major therapy for the ill."

A conditioner of what? Importantly, of your body's muscles, of which you have more than 600. These muscles are not for show —unless you are a professional "muscleman." They have a specific function in your body: they help you breathe and eat and, as we have seen, they help circulate the blood as well.

SETTING-UP EXERCISES?

These are well worth doing but most people find them dull and even fatiguing. If done in a group they can be somewhat more interesting, but the average man or woman does not usually stick to a program of such exercises for very long. Fortunately, most if not all of the benefits one derives from them are also obtainable from walking. Many of the same muscles—in the legs, the arms, the hips, the chest and elsewhere in the body—are exercised by walking as well as by setting-up exercises. And walking is much more enjoyable.

HOW YOU LOOK

If you make a habit of walking, you will soon get used to hearing people ask what you have been doing—you look different, seem younger and altogether more fit. And a glance in a full-length mirror will confirm this. As your stomach and back muscles develop, the middle-aged droop will disappear and your posture and all your movements will take on new authority and elasticity. People may not quite know in what way you look different, but they will be certain that you do. Moreover, the physical improvement cannot help but be accompanied by a corresponding improvement in your mental attitude. The apprehensive, nervous glance of the person who distrusts his body gives way to the confident look of the physically fit. If you feel this is an overstatement, think of one of your friends who takes pride in his body and of another who thinks of his body as a source of pain, trouble or illness.

87

A JOKE?

The story is told of the newly rich lady coming out of a luxury hotel followed by an attendant carrying her eight-year-old son in his arms. An acquaintance stops her and remonstrates that unless she gives the boy a chance to walk he will never learn how. The lady eyes her acquaintance haughtily. "Thank God he'll never have to," she sniffs.

Too many Americans these days are figuratively thanking God for not having to walk. Instead, they should be rendering thanks that they *can* walk. If, by some chance, they were rendered incapable of doing so, they would very soon consider the ability to walk one of the most precious gifts vouchsafed to man. But as man is constituted, he values least what he already has. It is only when he is deprived of it that he recognizes what it is worth.

NOT A CURE-ALL—BUT ALMOST

Most of us are sophisticated enough to laugh at the old advertisements for medicines or mechanical devices that promised cures for every known physical ailment from the common cold to cancer. So today, even though we are aware of the overall efficacy of walking, we are frequently reluctant to make specific claims. Yet, we can state confidently that the person who walks regularly may find that his exercise improves an arthritic condition or asthma. Besides strengthening the heart, it can also be helpful to diabetics and to persons with emphysema. And the improved muscle tone and development can help reduce or eliminate the various aches and pains in the lower and upper back that often result from weak muscles. Furthermore, exercise, especially walking, can alleviate that widespread and most stubborn complaint, hypochrondria. Get the man who thinks he is sick to know he is well, and you have done him just about the biggest favor there is.

18/Balance

One caution: no matter how excellent the results of your walking are, don't become one of those fanatics who build their life around a hobby or any other kind of pursuit. Especially, do not make it your sole topic of conversation. We all know the individual who talks endlessly about the state of his health, the food that agrees with him, the food that disagrees with him, the miracle doctor he has just found after twenty other doctors turned out to be quacks and money grubbers, and so on. A virtue can be turned into a vice by this kind of excess.

This may seem like strange advice coming from someone who has devoted a book, however small, to the subject of walking, but there is a difference. The purpose of this book is to enlist readers in an effort to avoid the ills that come from lack of sensible exercise. Once *you* have avoided these ills, you are not called on to be a voice in the wilderness—unless, of course, you want to write a book. Try hard not to be that deadliest of bores—the health bore.

CLUBS?

Many years ago, in simpler times, one New York City morning newspaper regularly carried announcements of a walking club that met every Sunday morning for a long walk through attractive country or to an interesting destination. Week after week, as many as 50 walkers, young and middle-aged, met to enjoy these walks. Now and then someone would drop out and a new face would be seen. The group as a whole was as healthy and happy an aggregation as you could find. Is such a club feasible today? It might be

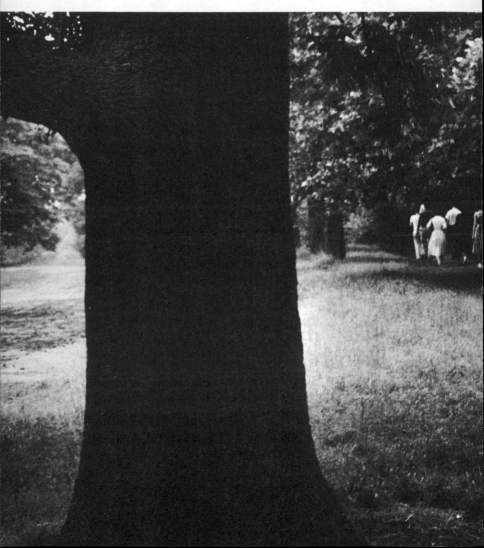

worth some reader's while to look into the matter.

PEDOMETERS?

We have nothing against pedometers but we do not believe they are essential to enjoyable walking. If you are determined to know how far you have walked, you can pick up a pedometer in most sporting equipment stores for under $10. Pedometers, by the way, are not quite as simple or accurate as a watch, and a balky one can introduce irritation into what could be a pleasant walk.

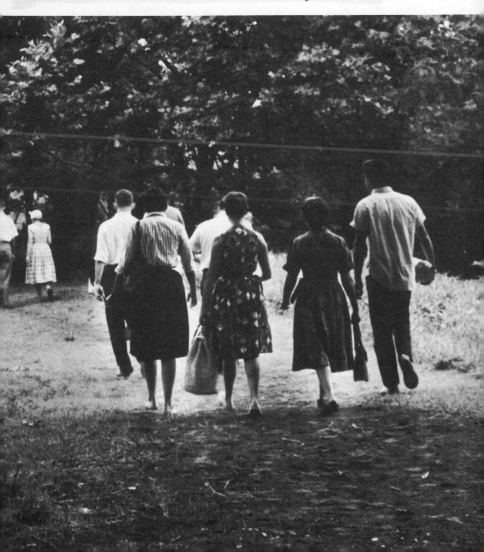

19/At the Bottom of It All

The most eloquent spellbinder in the world—he could be a combination of William Jennings Bryan and Winston Churchill—could not persuade you to walk if your feet hurt. And aching feet are almost as common in our country as aching backs. The American Podiatry Association has some suggestions you may find beneficial:

1) Take proper care of your feet by practicing regular, daily foot hygiene.

2) Exercise your feet and legs to promote circulatory exchange. This is most effective in the evening after a hard day. One such exercise: Elevate your feet, flex toes for about one minute, stopping as soon as the foot becomes pale. Allow feet to dangle down for one minute. Following this, keep legs in horizontal position for one minute. Repeat this entire procedure 10 times.

3) Use proper chairs and stools to avoid or at least to interrupt periods of standing during the day. Standing in one position for long periods contributes to stagnation of circulation.

4) Elevate the feet at various times during the day. This helps improve circulation.

5) Use floor mattings of different kinds to provide different resiliencies.

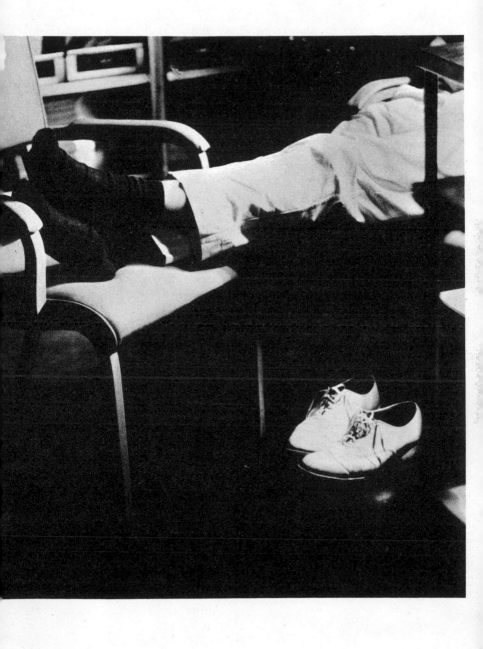

6) Alternate shoes at the office and at home. Constant use of high heels produces foot and leg changes which contribute a great deal to foot fatigue. If you're going to use high heels, a selection of shoes with varying heel heights will provide a necessary change.

7) Soak your feet after a day's work, followed by hot and cold sprays and a good foot powder. Some foot lotions are refreshing.

Podiatrists, who see a lot of infected and therefore hurting feet, advise that you trim your toe nails straight across and not shorter than the flesh. If you cut into the flesh at the corner of the toe you help solve the germs' housing problem. Their idea of the perfect home is one in a moist, dark, airless setting. Also watch out for blisters caused by improperly fitted shoes or torn shoe linings. The blessings of modern antibiotics and other powerful germ fighters make infections less dangerous than they were in the past—but those of us who are past 50 can still remember a United States President whose son died of an infected blister on his foot.

We also hear from podiatrists that they encounter some fantastic bunions and other foot malformations—many of them on women who cannot bring themselves to ask a shoe salesman for an honest size nine but insist on squeezing into a size six or seven. These would-be Cinderellas should be told that the day of princes and golden slippers is over and that even the Chinese no longer bind their girl children's feet to keep them tiny.

We are fully aware that the above paragraph is an exercise in futility. In all recorded history nobody has been able to cope successfully with the vanity of women.

THE PRESIDENT'S COUNCIL

One of the most influential bodies in the field of health education is the President's Council on Physical Fitness. This is what the Council recommends: *Walk—every chance you get.*

Walking, the Council declares, deserves special emphasis because "Walking is actually one of the best all-around physical activities. The massaging action the leg muscles exert on the veins as you walk improves the flow of blood back to the heart; when you walk you're improving not only your leg muscles but also the pumping action they provide. Walking costs nothing; there are many possible daily opportunities for it, and it can be enjoyable. Develop a brisk step, breathe deeply, swing your arms."

The Council has no axe to grind except that of making Americans fitter. If it says walking deserves special emphasis, should you not give it that emphasis?

WHO ELSE?

If there is one organization that has more information about health in all its aspects than any other non-medical group, that organization is the Metropolitan Life Insurance Company. That is why we find such Metropolitan pronouncements as these especially significant:

- A brisk daily walk can be a great help in taking off weight —and keeping it off.
- Exercise does not have to be either laborious or time consuming. One of the simplest ways is to make it a point to walk when you do not absolutely have to ride.
- Walking is a fine way to keep yourself in good shape.
- Remember you do not have to overdo to get results.
- Moderate exercise every day will help your body burn up superfluous fat, firm up muscles and smooth down bulges. And it will *not* increase your appetite.
- Moderate exercise appears to help protect against hypertension and coronary heart disease.

And a final word from the President's Council:

"Recent studies seem to indicate that lack of physical activity is more often the cause of overweight than is overeating."

Flying in the face of such authorities as these may be a bold act—but it is not the kind of exercise we recommend. Remain on terra firma, keep your feet moving, and stay alive!